Unbreakable Thoughts

Your Thoughts Become Things

Chapter 1

Intro

When you hear the question, "what is the mind?" what do you think of? Do you think of your actual brain? Or maybe even your thoughts? Do you immediately wonder deeply how the mind may work? The reality is all those things combined creates "the mind". You must understand how the brain works in order to use the power of your mind to your full advantage. People often underestimate how much power we have at the tips of your fingers, or the top of your head.

We have all heard the saying "Sticks and stones may break our bones, but words will never hurt me." While words can cause harm, it is true that most of our physical bodies can be broken out minds just do not break as easily. Especially our thoughts. When we understand fully what our brains and minds and even thoughts are capable of, we can not only change our lives, but we can change the world.

In this book, you will begin to deeply understand how to invest in your mind, manifestation, over coming obstacles, and how all these things connect to the unbreakable mind. While some of this might sound like foreign concepts at first, once you finish this book, you will be an expert. So, buckle up and get ready to fully immerse your mind, and reach the potential resting inside of you.

Chapter 2: How the Brain Works

We know the basics of the brain. It is inside of your head, more so, in your skull. But do you know what all it does? All the parts of the brain? The brain holds our thoughts, memories, our senses, helps us to move our bodies, and assists in controlling all our behaviors, even those like speaking and lying. The brain is the be-all, end-all of how humans exist and who humans are in its entirety.

As scientific as it might be, it is important to understand the parts of the brain and how they do what they do, to make us who we are and why we behave the way we do.

Certain parts of the brain control functions like breathing and pumping blood in and out of the heart. Some parts of the brain also control our bodily movement. A well-known part of the brain is the cerebellum. This particular part of the brain is what helps you to keep a beat to music or even perfect your jump shot, and volleyball serve.

The cerebrum is the part of the brain you will access in order to see memories you have stored, your intellectual ability, how you plan birthday parties and even how you manage your very busy schedule. This is the same part of the brain that allows us to remember those we have met before in passing and how close we were to that person. Next time you sit down with all your friends to play a board game you will be using the cerebrum for all of what is going on. Those people, the way you feel about them, even how you win the game every single time. This part of the brain is split in two, but they work together like a well-oiled machine.

One of the more commonly well-known parts of the brain is the frontal lobe. This is the part of the brain I mentioned previously about planning your schedule. This section will also be the location that all your short-term thoughts are stored.

Have you ever bitten into food and immediately feel a burning sensation, or taste a plethora of flavor? You might think it is just because of your mouth or the taste buds on your tongue. While these are a factor, your parietal lobes are actually the reason for these reactions. If you have an aversion to spice or a distain for certain textures, this part of the brain is what triggers that as well.

The occipital lobe is probably what you think. Its name is a bit of a giveaway. This is the part of the brain that processes images. When you see photos, colors, light. All these images are processing through this section of the brain. If this part of the brain is damaged or injured in anyway, it is what could cause blindness without direct damage being done to the eye.

The temporal lobe handles the processing sound. Your favorite song, the tune that is stuck in your head, the noise that you hear as you are sitting on the train, all of these must process through this lobe. It plays a direct role in all your other senses as well.

The brain also controls other feelings such as adrenaline, anger, and unhappiness. These are all controlled by the hypoth alamus.

While some of these terms might seem intimidating, just think of the brain as a giant computer. It has lots of nerves, tissue, and fatty deposits. It might just be a giant blob, but in reality, it holds much more power than even what we realize. Chemicals move through the brain collects information and so much more.

Do you think you have any control over this? Do you feel like you have a say over what happens in your mind? Do you have the power to change the chemicals in your mind? The answer you might think is no, but the real answer is yes. You have much more say over all of this than you think.

Now that you have heard the scientific understanding of at least some of the brain, it in its entirety would take a whole book, we can dive into the more metaphysical side of the mind to understand just how unbreakable your mind really is.

Chapter 3: The Power of the Mind:

While we learned before that the mind can make our bodies move, storing our memories, planning a future, and even processing photos – it is even more powerful than any of that. Even your thoughts alone are more powerful than that. As strong as your thoughts are, is exactly as strong as you are. Your mind has the power to control everything that may happen in your future. We will progress deeper as the book progresses forward; however, you must know that you need to be more careful of what you think. If you replay failures repeatedly in your mind, you will only ever experience failure. If the loop in your mind, is that you will always struggle finically, you will never know the finical freedom you deserve. You must first think the thoughts you want to come to life. That is merely the beginning.

Like any power, or ability, you must train and make it stronger. Nothing develops overnight. This is going to take time and effort. You will even be able to uplift and help those around you as well. Who does not want to help their friends? Planting seeds that will grow is only one part of what you will be able to do with your mind.

When you first start this whole process, it might feel like daydreaming. In reality, it is what you will be doing to some degree. You must think about exactly what you want, desire, and deserve. Have you ever seen yourself accomplishing all your goals? You need to. You must believe exactly what you are thinking about. If you are working on starting a podcast, envision yourself posting your first episode. See your followers increasing. Look at yourself as a successful now. While you might not see it day one, it will start to come into reality. Not only will your behaviors start to become your real life, but you will also start creating better habits surrounding all your goals.

Many people use these abilities as a way to obtain better health, higher wealth, work promotions, and even open businesses. You can even use these powers to become stronger in relationships. Work on rejecting those negative thoughts that so easily come to your mind. It is easier to be negative than positive. Positivity, that is harder to come by. Those are the things you must fight for. At some point in your life, I am sure you have heard the connection of the glass half full or half empty. It is easy to think harshly, however pushing yourself to think happier thoughts and more positively will pay off in ten folds. It is time to start seeing that glass as half full, always, in every situation.

People underestimate our speech and how we talk. Body language and words hold power. It is why so many businesses use slogans and catch phrases. We forget how much we care about words when we use them so often and without thinking about it. If your spouse says, "hey can you come help me with the chores?" your reaction will be much gentler than if they say, "will you get up and do something about this pile of dishes?" If you want those around you to choose their words wisely, should it not first start with you?

As much power as our words have, we also have the power of suggestion in other people's lives. At times, we mention things and they hold weight, without us even meaning for them to. It could be because of who we are speaking to. Our friends are going to care about our opinions more than a stranger will. However, sometimes our words carry weight regardless of who we are speaking to. So, the next time you are about to tell someone to "quit their dead-end job" or to "dump their lame partner" remember that those suggestions may carry more weight than you intended and could cause hurt that you did not mean to inflict. If the job isn't really that terrible or the person isn't actually bad for them, maybe tread lightly on the verbal messages.

The power of the mind is a creative power. It is not something you can hold in your hand or see laying on the floor. Yet, it is very real. The more you learn to manage these thoughts and harness the power of your mind the more tangible it will become. We will dive deeper into how to access the power of your mind as we get further in this book, and as you learn more, the more real it will become.

Chapter 4: Investing in Your Mind

When it comes to investing in your mind, you must invest in yourself as a whole. You will need to make sure you are doing everything you can to better your future. You have to build you knowledge, confidence, purpose, and increase your wealth. You need to set some achievable goals for yourself. Make a list of all these goals. You might need to budget your funds accordingly even. Financial freedom come with work and might even require you to be a bit of a penny pincher. If you have looming debt, get it all paid off. That might be your amazon credit card or your mom that you borrowed $200 from weeks ago. While your mom might not be able to report to the credit bureau, having any looming debt is not going to do you any justice in becoming any level of free. While you are working on debts and your financials, start saving money. This can be in the form of investments or even a savings account. Somehow, you must start saving some money.

Have you ever considered how you will plan your future or what that will look like? Have you considered furthering your education? Maybe that is not going back to college but, you should never stop learning. Keep expanding your horizons, learn a new trade even. Keeping new information flowing, is a great way to build who you are and your mind.

While working on your mind, you might also want to consider working on your vessel. Start working out. Start eating better. Take your vitamins. Yes, every single day you need to take those vitamins. Go outside, even when it's a bit cold. Realign with nature. Touch earth and balance your body to balance your mind.

Do you have a passion that could be monetarily lucrative? You need to start a side hustle. You can do something more tangible like door dash or start selling those paintings that you have hidden from the world. Whatever you love, whatever you are good at, start making some money off it, outside of your 9-5, as you still need to keep that.

With all these investments in yourself, be realistic. Be real and do not be hard on yourself. You will stumble but you will see immediate change in your life. Even if those changes are small. So now, you have invested in yourself, how do you start to fully invest in your mind?

Something to keep in mind is that your mind is a direct reflection of yourself and your life. If your life is chaotic and messy, your mind will be as well. Humans thrive on knowledge. It is exactly why you are reading this book. It is time that you get back on track and start to really understand just how unbreakable your mind is.

Do you value yourself? If you do not, you can expect that no one else will either. Place value, first in yourself and what you can do and handle. Mentally, physically, and emotionally. Feed your mind. Study new information and learn some new skills. Dissect some of the stuff that you already know, is there anything that you can explore further? Develop what you can within yourself, determine what new things you can add to your personal vault of information.

What is your truest purpose in life? Find your inner peace first. If you are not mentally calm, you can expect that you will stumble more. Calm the noise and listen to what your path is. Meditate, reflect on what appears to you while meditating. Do you wish to be an author? Start a podcast? Own your own business? Don't allow yourself to become hopeless any longer. While big dreams can seem far away, we are both here because we are learning just how powerful our minds are. Hopelessness will only lead to negative thoughts. Once you find the purpose inside of you; latch onto that. This will be the start of what is to come and be the why every time you start to doubt that you can handle this.

Do you remember back in grade school before a big test teachers would remind you as often as they could to eat a well-balanced breakfast and get plenty of rest? We talked about feeding your body what it needs, so let's target that sleep portion of that advice. Without great sleep, your mind will not work properly. Not only will a lack of sleep create a chemical imbalance in your brain it can also be a cause of anxiety, depression, mood swings, and more. Get a new bed, set alarms for going to sleep and waking up, avoid unnecessary naps and start making your sleep a priority. Your body but more importantly your mind, will thank you.

As cliché as it might be, start picking up more books. Reading will develop your mental state but can also regulate your emotional aliments as well. Reading can lower anxiety, help with depression, and reduce stress. I mentioned it before, but sleep is critical as well and reading before bed will increase your sleep patterns in a positive way as well.

When is the last time you learned a new hobby? As mundane as it might seem, it really increases your brain and mental development. Do not just learn one; learn several. Do not settle for just one. Once you have perfected one new hobby, take on another one. Don't ever stop learning new things, it is going to be critical to feeling better about yourself by building your self esteem but will also help you to feel competent.

When is the last time you sat down alone and had a quiet moment to yourself? If you can not remember, it has been too long. You need start making this a priority as well. Meditation is a great way to turn off your mind and the outside noise, and really look within. Check out my book, *Mindfulness Meditation* to learn all the ways to make meditation apart of your routine. Meditation can help you sleep which in turns, provides you with more energy. Breathing methods and many other ways to meditate will drastically improve your life and your mind in amazing ways.

Humans need interactions with other people. No matter how much of an introvert you are or how great alone time might feel, you must spend time with other people. People go to extreme measures to be apart of a community that they feel comfortable or accepted in. Isolation will cause severe mental disorders, for even the sanest of minds. You must keep your mind sharp in order to fully understand just how unbreakable your thoughts are. Being social will keep you in line and push you to sleep well, learn new skills, and take on new experiences. Studies have shown that maintaining social lives will even help you live longer, no matter how long you live, having people you care about around will absolutely make your life fuller.

Declutter and organize your home and office space. Start with one room at a time. Remove unnecessary items that take up space and gather dust. If you have the funds, revamp, and redecorate each room as you go. If you can not do that, at least deep clean each space, and remove all the items that no longer serve a purpose any longer. Once you have deep cleaned and simplified each space in your home you need to create a cleaning schedule to keep up on your space. Only you know your ability and what days make sense to do what things. You can choose to do a room a day, or certain tasks on certain days. Whatever is going to work best to ensure that you can keep up on the chores in your space. Keeping a clean and organized space will rid your mind of clutter. Having a space full and unorganized will make your mind feel just like that as well. Having a space reflective of order will help you feel more in control and growing toward all the goals you have set for yourself.

Have you ever heard the saying "you are only as strong as your weakest link."? This saying is even true when talking about yourself. You will never be able to achieve your strongest potential, without knowing exactly what your weaknesses are. You must look within yourself and stare into your greatest inabilities. We all have things that we just are not great at. Look directly into those things and do your best to use them in the opposite way and to your advantage. For example, if you are not great at art – keep drawing. Even if you never show anyone, keep pushing yourself to do those scary things even if you feel like it is impossible, and you are doomed to fail. You will get better, and that is going to make you feel stronger by the moment.

While you are focusing on your lesser strengths, work on ridding yourself of some of your less than great habits. If you bite your fingernails, research how to stop. If you drink several sodas a day, cut down and eventually stop drinking it altogether. Bad habits are hard to break but you will feel better once you have gotten rid of some of those habits. Plus, clearing your mind of certain things will open it up to learn and explore new habits, such as reading or yoga!

Are you someone who stays comfortable in repeating the same day to day behaviors? Well, it is time to break that cycle as well. It is time to start taking some risks. While this could be in life, maybe it is even your job. Have you ever heard of a "yes day"? While this is often something parents do for children to encourage them to get to enjoy a day free of their nay saying parents, maybe YOU need a yes day. This would be a day saying yes to all those things that you would normally say no to, out of habit or fear. Take the leap. The reward might end up being the best thing that ever happened, just by taking a risk.

While just above I mentioned saying yes more, you must also learn when to say no. Do you have friends or family members that tend to push your boundaries and make you do things you have made clear you are not okay with? People will take advantage of those who have a hard time standing their ground or defending themselves. Create those boundaries but this time, stick to them. Maybe it is your habit of lending money and never expecting repayment or running errands for them when you are far to busy to actually do it. It is time to say no and mean it. Follow through with those lines. You will feel better because of it.

When all else fails, and you feel like all the above is too far out of your reach, never be too egotistical to ask for help. Find a mentor. This could be someone in your personal life that you look up to or someone professionally who you think could help you grow as a person. Having someone to reach out to and rely on when you face hard decisions will only benefit you in the long run. Work on talking to them about why their mentoring would be helpful to you. Some people have several mentors, so they can target all the points of growth that you might need. Use their strengths to grow your own. It is not wrong to reach out and ask for help from those who can provide it.

Now that you have all the resources you need to invest in your mind; we can keep going to further your growth and to really unlock all the power you have within!

Chapter 5: State of Mind

Conscious, Unconscious, and Subconscious

We have broken down the brain and all the details of what information is held where. Now, we need to dive a bit deeper into the parts of the mind, that maybe are less heard of or not even known of. These are the things that you cannot see or touch or even that scientists do not have as much information on. The information we are going to dive into can be broken down into 3 well know states of mind; the conscious, subconscious, and the unconscious mind. Some things we are hyper aware of, others, not so much. Let's break these down.

The conscious state of mind explains our behaviors, through process and awareness in decision making. The subconscious state of mind is our actions and response to events we encounter in life. The unconscious state of mind defines all the deep memories that we may or may not bury deep within. We might not even be aware that these exist, but they do. In every single one of us.

The conscious is the state of mind most commonly known. It is what makes us different than other animals or beings. Being able to respond with thoughts is what makes it conscious. We are taking in information constantly; our conscious mind works on over drive to ensure that we are aware of what is going on around us. It is the easiest states of mind to understand as it is our daily processing abilities.

On the other hand, the unconscious mind goes deeper than most realized. We dove into the scientific understandings of the brain, but science cannot completely understand the unconscious state of mind. Some have tried to pull out the deeper repressed thoughts we have buried, often used to help those with trauma. Much of those deeper thoughts can lead to issues in the future. These unconscious thoughts will surface later in life, usually in bad habits, fears, and even recurring cycles. If we leave our unconscious mind unchecked and unaccounted for, we will make minor mistakes, and sometimes larger ones. Many companies are training on unconscious bias. We easily fall into behaviors and habits of how we speak, leading to leud or offensive behaviors. While these behaviors are accidental and habit, there might be deeper meaning to them. Getting to the bottom of the unknown feelings are critical, so start doing some internal work to see if the slips in thoughts and behaviors that are just that or are they some deep hidden trauma.

The subconscious state of mind is often explained as a protective layer so we are not overloaded with all the feelings that might be thrown at us on a daily basis. "The mind forgets nothing". No matter how forgetful the mind might be, in reality, we store most things. You might have an over-working subconscious if you tend to forget things easily. It stores the stuff that we need to survive our everyday lives and even stores information that we do not use every day but that we still need. Riding our bike, typing without looking, how to tie our shoes. No matter how long we go without riding out bike or tying our shoes our minds will do these things without thought. Think of this state of mind as when we go into autopilot. In those moments we behave without thought. What we must keep in mind is that we have the power to change even our subconscious.

There are times that we create habits and they become actual habits. For example, say you have always written your 8's as an infinity sign, sideways. You recently started doing 2 circles stacked on top of each other. At first, you had to work for it. You had to make yourself change the way you wrote it. Now, however, when you write it, it happens entirely without thought. It is going to feel like that is how you have always written it. There are times that we can resist change at times, due to our subconscious. We need to push past these barriers and strive for change. Change is what will help you to unlock your minds full potential and build on its already unbreakable foundation.

The 3 states of mind can seem very separate, but they all rely on each other. You need each of them to process properly and make decisions that we make. We do, however, need to tap into all 3 states of mind and be working on things to improve our overall mental health and strength. Meditation is a great way to tap into that deeper awareness. All the ways mentioned in the investing in your mind section will help to clear some of the brain fog that we get naturally with our ever-changing states of mind.

Chapter 6: Philosophies

We spoke a bit about our unconscious and subconscious states of mind, and even our conscious state of mine. It only makes sense to dive into some great philosophies, they are really the basis of a lot of the topic that we will or have covered in this book. While there are so many philosophers and philosophies so we will not be able to cover all of them, I do think touching on them is important.

Have you ever heard the name Sigmund Freud? He started his research as a neurologist and was able to make connections in mental illness to the study of the brain. He was also able to help tons of people and a lot of his ideas are still present in mental health environments. Prior to Freud, scientists and doctors did not think there was a way to help those with mental disorders. He was the first person to really dive into the 3 states of mind we talked about before, and the correlation that they had with each other. Freud also dove deeply into the human's ego. He talked a lot about our defensiveness when someone confronts us, or we are faced with a difficult topic. Generally, the reason we become defensive is because our ego. We will discuss the ego further later in this book.

Freud is also the originator of the practice of therapy we use in modern medicine, one on one therapy which is based on us talking through our issues or things we might be facing that is causing us problems in our mental health. He was also known for talking about fixation as well. Becoming obsessed with something or latching onto it. This can create bad habits and could keep those habits going our entire lives.

One of the coolest things that Freud was apart of understanding dreams. He correlated our dreams to our unconscious mind. He considered dreams a peephole into thing we otherwise would not know. He strongly believed that our dreams were the way we could achieve our deepest desire, all the things that our ego will get in the way of. I advise that you start logging your dreams now! Study them after you have logged them, you might be shocked by what you realized you want or need.

Have you ever been in a situation where someone immediately denied or rationalized something they had be apart of? This could be reasons and excuses as to why they will not leave a relationship or push for a promotion they are due for at work. This is another thing that Freud talked a lot about, why we justify behaviors and choices rather then facing these things and making some change. Freud had many other theories where he focused on women and even religion. Look into him and see what other ideas he impacted for modern day life.

When speaking of Freud and philosophies there are a few others that need recognized as well. Heinz Kohut was another philosopher that is important to talk about. Kohut was most known for his idea focusing on self-psychology, which is essentially focused on narcissistic personalities. His main belief system was that narcissists were created by unempathetic parents. They were not watered properly by those they looked up to or taught how to build their own self esteem.

Another well-known philosopher was Carl Jung. He was known for analytical psychology. He often spoke of the unconscious mind as well as psychotherapy. Freud was even intrigued by Jung's ideas and these two brilliant men worked closely for years. They did eventually go their separate ways as person visons did not align with one another.

Jung conceptualized the idea of introversion and extraversion. Most people will label themselves as one or the other. Extraverts are generally people who are outgoing, energetic, and often the center of attention. Where an introvert is someone who is reserved, often falling to the background in a social setting. These attitude types are commonly used but people don't always know that they might fluctuate. Which umbrella do you fall under most often, extravert or introvert? Since we are developing the mind, it would benefit you to know which of these you are most often. Understanding this about your self can help develop behavior patterns. As an extravert you might have to develop the ability to know when to let others take the spotlight. As an introvert, you must start pushing yourself to more limits and come out of the safe bubble that is your mind and silence. It will greatly benefit your mind to push yourself out of your norms and dive deeper into Jung's ideas.

While there are mounds of more information on these philosophers as well as others, we do not have the time to explain everyone and all their perspectives. These 3 have some great correlation all we are studying and learning to develop in this book, and it would benefit you to do some research on them and see which of these, or maybe someone not listed, to see who your heart is most drawn to. See which ideas and thoughts speak to you the most. Always keep in mind, you might only resonate with only one person's ideas, you might see perspectives of several and their connections.

Chapter 7: Placebo Effect

Have you ever tricked yourself into believe something? Taken a drink that helped cure an aliment? Reminded yourself of the concept – "use it or lost it" and said that if you walked a mile a week it would keep you young? Anything that you have said repeatedly only for it to come true? These are a few examples of the placebo effect. The placebo affect is all about connecting the mind to the body. While "believe it" will not cure cancer, it will make you feel better whether that be sleeping, eating, or even pain.

Placebo will increase dopamine; in turn it will immediately change the emotional state of mind. We must tread lightly with how aware we are that we are almost "tricking" our mind and body. Remember, you have to believe it for it work. Just like a mantra, repeat to yourself that it does work and eventually it will. Doctors have used placebo to test drugs and their effectiveness.

While you can use the placebo effect in the medical studies, you can also use it to encourage your mind into healthier behaviors that you will later use to create the space and ability to build on your unbreakable thoughts. Studies have shown that placebo effect can help people who suffer from anxiety, fatigue and even how rapid your heart races. Using a mantra can really benefit your mental state in those high stress moments. This in turn will strengthen your mind and build your thoughts.

Remind yourself that your mind can not be broken. It can not be damaged. Your thoughts are your strength, and you alone have the power to develop them and build them up. Use the placebo effect to challenge yourself and keep telling yourself that you will succeed and that your thoughts are going to change not only your life but those closest to you.

Chapter 8: Negative Thoughts

While the placebo effect is extremely powerful; so is negative thinking. While the simple idea is that you have to push yourself to be more positive, it goes beyond that. Sometimes our negative thinking can prepare is for what is to come. Usually someone who thinks of the bad before the good can navigate a path out of it before it even hits. You can not let the negative thoughts take over, however use them to your full advantage if they are not something you are able to rid yourself of. The common theme of this books is going to be just that – using things you already possess to your advantage and to understand the power of your own mind.

When you have already predetermined what might go wrong, you aren't often going to be caught off guard. For example, if you think negatively and you are walking into a job interview, you might think "they won't hire me" – thus you will be more authentic and more for yourself, being exactly the perfect fit for the role. This can work with positive thinking of course as well, be confident and sure of yourself when walking in and the same outcome is likely to happen.

Even children tend to succumb to their negative thinking. When a child is craving attention, they will process all the ways to achieve that. They will choose negative behaviors from those negative thoughts because any attention, even bad, is better than none. To the best of their ability, they are using negative thoughts to their advantage, and you should as well.

Start working on stopping your hyper fixation. When something bad happens do not let it ruin your entire day. If one rude comment from a stranger can dictate your entire mood and the rest of your day you are not using that negative energy to your advantage. You must hear it, feel it, see it. You can not change what the stranger did but you can change what you do next, with those negative feelings. Do the opposite of what that stranger did. When you pass another stranger, be extra kind to them. Go out of your way to uplift them

The next time you and your partner argue instead of thinking "they are so rude, all they do is pick at me" or "they never see all that I do for them", remind yourself of what you truly feel for them. Do not gaslight yourself obviously. If your partner is horrible to you, let them go. But if you only think these things after a normal relationship hiccup; instead try to think about all the wonderful things your partner does for you. "They are so kind and caring" or "they treat me with such love and compassion", even "they truly have my best interest at heart". Not only will this strengthen the love you have for your partner, but it will also strengthen your mind.

We are all hard wired at birth essentially to reflect and latch onto any thing negative that comes our way when we need to feel and see those and immediately turn them into something beneficial to you. You must stop self-deprecating and self-sabotaging. Start to see the good in all those moments that feel so dark. Reshape and use the placebo effect, to create new patterns that will change your future and the path you are following.

Be sure to bask in those moments of happiness as well. Replay those joyous moments on repeat. Be aware that you will never be able to make those negative moments go away. It is going to exist, no matter what. You just must do whatever you need to un order to use even the worst moments to make you stronger than you were the day before. Most importantly, never let those bad days, ruin all the good that remains.

Chapter 9: Using You Mind to Overcoming Obstacles

There are so many things that we can do to face what we are bound to have to deal with, but do not fret. There are so many ways to overcome the unknown and what is going to come your way!

You first need to realize that appreciation is important. Appreciate the small things and when a when is a win, let it be just that. Step outside of the immediate doom and gloom that is easy to fall into and start to be grateful of all the small things that surround you and make you who you are.

Have you ever been asked, "what is your biggest fear?" What is your response? Do you say death, spiders, or heights? Some fears are not as easily faced; however, some are. You need to face the ones that you can. Run into the storm of your worst fear. Start taking risks and jump from the plane, go bungee jumping, or go hold a tarantula. You are going to feel like the walls are closing in around you but take some deep breathes and face it! After all, your mind will feel stronger than ever after you have faced that fear that has been holding you back.

Keep a positive mindset. We are going to dive deeper into complaining later but remember the weight your words and complaints have. Hold those complaints close to your chest. When you are going on a hike with your partner and you despise hiking, the heat, the bugs, the aching body, and the constant urge to sit down – remember who you are there for and why you are doing it. Connect with nature and smile at your partner, they will be happier than you could imagine. Refrain from blabbing that you are so miserable, or you might ruin a great experience with someone that you love.

While giving yourself grace is hard to do at times, you have to. Be kind to yourself through every single phase of growth because there will be some slip ups. You must be gentle. You have been through so much. While being gentle you need to be real with yourself. Sometimes what we think we need is exactly the opposite. What is needed will happen, no matter what.

In this world it is so easy to get caught up in what others are doing and trying to do better or one up everyone around you. Comparing yourself to others comes naturally. Especially with access to the internet now. Your journey and path might be very different than someone else. While it might take you longer than others or in a more difficult way. You will get there when the time is right or you. No one likes a one-upper. When you are talking about how rough your day was and your friends undermines your feelings by saying you had it easy compared to them, it is not a good feeling. Do not be that person, ever. Go out of your way to listen and be there actively when someone else is expressing their hardships. Be a good person even when just speaking to those around you and in your inner circle.

There comes a moment during any phase of change when you might realize enough is enough. You are learning when you let go and it's a good thing you are. This does not mean to let go of the goal. That should never come unless the goal shifts. However, you need to learn to let go of all the things that do not serve you anymore. It is time to keep only the things that provide a benefit to you and your life. If your job is weighing you down, find a new one. If your family is pushing you into a corner or triggering your negative energy or treating you like a black sheep, draw a line in the sand and create a boundary. Protect what makes your life better and remove what continues to cause you grief. It is time you put YOU first. Without any doubt and with great intention set to back all your choices.

Chapter 10: Overcoming Fears

Briefly in another chapter we talked about facing fears. We need to take a bit of a deeper dive. Facing your fears is a great way to strengthen your mind.

The first thing you need to do is breathe. I mentioned it before, you will feel like the walls are closing in around you. You are going to want to hyperventilate. You must slow down your breathing and do some counting. Apple watches will now ask you to do deep breathing exercises every now and then. You can start working on this now on your own without the watch, so you are ready when that rapid breathing takes over. So, walk toward that fear and breathe. You might stumble, especially at first, you might even walk away and not be able to face it right away but keep pushing and keep walking toward the things that you are afraid of.

Even though it might seem scary, you must imagine the worst-case scenario. What is going to happen if you get on the plane? Or when you are walking on that very high bridge? Envision the worst thing that could happen. This is going to prepare you for anything that may come. You must see the worst so when it does not happen you can take a deep breathe and start to feel better. Once you see that your deepest fears are not as likely to happen as you thought, your fears will not feel as big.

Perfection is impossible. Remember that and stop striving for perfection. Things are hard enough, do not add to the pressure of it all by trying to accomplish something that you never will, perfection. You need to be real with yourself and what is to come. Perfection is not going to exist, and it shouldn't. If you were to ever be "perfect" – how would you ever know what to keep striving for? Would you finally feel complete once you are perfect? If so, you will have nothing more to strive for, but we are never really finished being better. No matter how close we are to being the person we want, there is always more work to be done. Not only are you never going to achieve that level of perfection, but you are also going to drive yourself mad trying. Realize that "perfect" is exactly what you need and exactly where you are headed as every version of your self is the most perfect version that it can be.

One thing that is often underestimated is talking when something scares you. Talking about your fears will weaken them. Speak to a friend or family member about all the things you fear. Say the words directly. Not only will it weaken the strength of the fear, but it will also make you see that you are stronger than you realize. Hearing the words "I am terrified of spiders. They are so small and have so many legs and are covered in hair." Might just make you see that you are bigger and scarier than any spider.

The most important step when facing your fears is going to be to reward yourself. As we talked about before, small wins are still wins. One tiny spider at a time. Small steps leading to big leaps. Next time you get through a hard time or face a fear and even stand near a spider without screaming and running take yourself out for dessert or to your favorite coffee shop. You earned it.

So, in order to strengthen your mind and really hone your powers you must first overcome the fears you have been hiding. They will hold you down and hold you back form the growth you are working so hard on. It is time to let those things go along with all the other stuff that no longer serves you. Do you see a bit of a trend in this book yet? You must first relinquish those things that will not allow you to become the best version of yourself, so that version can come to the surface.

Chapter 11: BDC

While seeing those letters might not mean anything to you just yet, they will. BDC

means Blame, Complain, and Defend. It is important to hear about BCD to understand

what affect it has on you and what parts if any, should you keep doing. There is never

really a time that you should BDC. Placing blame, complaining, or becoming defensive

will only lead you to your own demise.

It is easy to place blame on others when something bad happens. You burn your dinner, you are stuck in traffic, or you break your finger. The immediate reaction in any of these scenarios is to blame those around you. The person who pulled you away from the stove to help them while dinner cooked, the person with the flat tire in front of the long line of cars just trying to get home, or the person who threw you the football that stubbed your finer. None of these people or circumstances were intentional so avoid blaming them for your misfortune. It will only hold you back and keep you down in the dumps.

Complaining will do much of the same. We mentioned it before but by constantly complaining you are creaking a negative bubble around yourself. The next time you feel yourself slipping into the habit and wanting to complain go take a walk or make yourself some iced coffee. Do something that you love and enjoy. It will help you to lose the negative energy and dissipate the complaint before it ever leaves your lips.

As far as defending, we talked a bit about the philosophies around defensive mechanisms we all have. You must be careful with this. While defending yourself when being attached or disturbed is okay. It is defensiveness that is dangerous. It is common knowledge that when someone is defensive immediately, it is because they carry some form of guilt, or their ego is tarnished. Defensive behavior is derived from the ego. We will discuss the ego later but be mindful of it when you want to defend something without really understanding where the protectiveness comes from.

Once you start to rid yourself of the immediate urge to BDC you will see how much you did it, but you will also see how treacherous it has been to your mental growth. The power of your thoughts are directly from you. They begin and end with you and your behaviors. Stopping the bad habits and start creating your own future and best practices now. You will start to see exactly how strong your mind is.

Chapter 12: Protecting Your Mind

While we are working on building the strength of our minds and thoughts, we must protect our mind. If you can protect your mind from allowing the BCD behaviors, negative thoughts and even the unconscious minds you must take preventative measures. When your thoughts are pure, your intentions will be the foundation of the most of what we are doing through this book.

It might sound redundant but the link between our body and out mind is crucial. This does not mean go to the gym 5 days a week and working out for 5 hours a day. It just means that you must protect your body and energy, thus protecting your mental space. Life flows from inside of you. It is directly linked to your mind so what you feed it, what you process, and even how you treat yourself is all going to play a factor in exactly what you mind is subjected to. You have to push yourself to find inner peace. Not matter what you must find that safe space. Peace is going to give you the calm that you need to accomplish all your goals. When you start to feel those bad feelings of envy or malice, you must derail and work toward grounding yourself.

It is idea to be careful with how much you worry you carry with you. Worrying leads to only stress and anxiety. Take strides to rid yourself of those things that weigh you down.

Keep yourself in the moment as often as you can. Be aware of the right now. You can not push away the bad things that come, they are going to. It is life. Feel the feelings that those things bring but do not hold onto them. Let the feelings come and go, flow in and out. As fleeting as the moment is, let that sadness go away in that moment as well. Do your best to avoid taking that moment into the next with you.

When is the last time you did something nice for yourself? Took yourself to the spa, bought yourself something you wanted, or even just spent time doing something that you love? While protecting your mind, you must do things that you enjoy in order to get there. Too much work and not enough play will only lead you to a life of boredom and hardship. Your mind needs to be treated to things that make you whole and happy.

Have you ever heard the phrase "count your blessings"? It is true. You have to be grateful for what you have done and how far you have come. Count those blessings. Look at what you have completed so far and look at what you have completed and really give yourself a pat on the back. Without praise, how will you ever really feel like you accomplished anything. We might hear things from others, but you must also hear it from yourself as well.

Work toward protecting your mind and your progress will reflect it. In order to water and grow something you must first keep it from harms way. Do you know what is almost most harmful compared to other things? You and your ego. Let's dive into that next.

Chapter 13: Keeping Your Ego in Check

What is the first thing that you think of when you hear the word ego? Be definition it is a person's sense of self-esteem or feeling of self-importance. Your ego is how you interact with other people as well and even how well you connect with others. Egos are needed but keeping them in check and under wraps is just as important, in not just how you deal with others but also how they will deal with you. Keeping it in check is going to be critical to your growth and really allowing you to keep your thoughts unbreakable.

Something commonly said is "get over yourself" when someone feels like you are being egotistical. This is a rather harsh way of saying, "hey your ego is showing". We should be a tad bit full of ourselves but with grace and not with your ego being the leader in that feeling. You do not want to become arrogant when feeling sure of yourself. Arrogance equals danger, often hidden by our ego. Our ego is what will dissipate our empathy and that is never going to benefit you or those around you.

Have you ever been labeled as a control freak? If not, do you still feel that need to have a say in everything around you? I am sure we all feel it pertaining to certain things, whether that be money, cleaning, our kids, or maybe even relationships. You will have to learn to relinquish some of that need to control everything around you. You will always be faced with things that you just cannot control; this is life. Much like you can not stop negative things from happening at times, outside sources will play a factor and those are things we just can not control. The sooner you realize that the easier it will become to adjust when "bad" things come your way. The moment when something goes wrong, do you respond with "everything is ruined"? That is your ego. Do you often feel like everyone, even the universe is out to get you? Again, your ego. Try to embrace the moments of lack of control. Choose to allow someone else to take the reins, even when everything is screaming for you to jump back in.

Affirmations are key to keeping your ego in check. You might repeat positive things to yourself such as "everything is fine", "you are capable", or even "I can do whatever I set my mind to". It is likely that your ego is going to try and tell you otherwise as soon as you whisper those affirmations to yourself, but shut that voice down immediately., every single time.

Are you jaded? It is a weird question but seriously, are you? Did something happen to you years ago that you are holding onto and is it causing you to feel cold and shut off from happiness? Do you have a grudge against someone from your past? If the answer is yes to any of the above, it is time to let it go. Whether is be by confronting the issue or by forgiving it. Your ego keeps you holding onto the hate in your heart. Look with in and remember to avoid BDC. Pointing the finger or blaming something other than your ego is only going to lead you down a continued path of despair. Your ego is feeding that anger. This is not to say that everyone and every situation in your life must be forgotten or forgiven. Somethings just hurt deeper. You can still have boundaries and keep people at a distance, but forgiveness is inside of you.

While we are on the topic of forgiveness, have you forgiven yourself? We are humans, we are bound to have made some mistakes along the way. You will struggle to forgive others if you are still holding onto something that you did in the past. Everything that has happened or that you have done is a lesson. The good, the bad and the in between, are lessons to learn from. Take every mistake you have made and grow from them. When in doubt; ask for help with forgiving yourself. Maybe that is reaching out to someone you feel you wronged, or professional help. When you are struggling to see the lesson, ask someone. Outside eyes are a great tool for seeing things we might have blinded ourselves to.

In order to keep your ego in check start to listen more and learn as much as you can. Learning a new skill or being willing to do things you would not have considered in the past is a great way to keep your mind fresh and ego at a lull. Even if your reaction is "ewe", especially if your reaction is "ewe", do it. Maybe that is learning to ride a horse, or exercising more, do it without judgement. Those gut reactions of distaste are your ego. Shut it down. Keep your internal voice quiet, so your actual voice does not say something it might not mean. You do not know what you will love or enjoy if you have yet to experience it.

Start admitting when you are wrong, even if that is hard. Thinking that you are never wrong is breed and watered in the ego. Not a single person in this world is always right. So, be honest when you are wrong. Getting humbled, especially by yourself, is great for the soul. It really does something long term to the ego. So, allow yourself to be humbled and admit when you are wrong.

When push comes to shove, trust those people closest to you. Your best friend or life partner, likely knows all your secrets. With having that level of knowledge about you, they are likely to tell you about yourself when you are not able to do it yourself. You need that. We all do. You will need to be humbled with the truth, whether it comes from someone else or within you. That person or those people will be able to see when it is your ego talking easier than you might be able to see it, so listen to them.

Shutting down your ego might be one of the most difficult things you have had to do to date. However, it is going to be one of the most rewarding things for your mind. You need your mind strong, and your ego weakened. This is going to take time and continued work, so keep doing this, no matter what. 10 years from now, you will still be shutting your ego down at times and that is okay. It is something that is never ending.

Chapter 14: Motivation

Motivation at its core is the drive to do something. There is so much more to it than just that. Motivation is the combination of need, drive, incentive, and reward. These are all the phases of motivation.

The first phase is need. You must find a NEED for something to find any form of motivation. Let's use this example as we break this down. You need to renovate your bathroom. It is old and outdated and just does not fit your ever-changing style. You have found the need for change, but now you must find the DESIRE to get the job done. Jump on Pinterest and start looking at some inspirational bathrooms. Those pinned photos will now become your INCENTIVE. That is what you want it to look and feel like when you walk into that completed bathroom. You know when it is complete it is going to be a place that you love and be a better fit for who you are. The end results, well that, is your REWARD. You have the plan laid out and the motivation to get there.

How important is the goal to you? What happens if you start the project and do not follow through? Well, in this case, you will have a half-finished bathroom that may or may not even be functioning. Are you going to hate the room even more now that it is half complete? Staying motivated is important for so much more than just a remodel of a room in your home. In order to achieve any goals, you have set for yourself and in your life, even finishing this book, you will have to learn to stay motivated.

Setting realistic expectations is going to be key in not only staying motivated but also to accomplish the result you desire. Avoid timelines that you just can not meet. If you say, "I will have this bathroom finished in one weekend" you are setting yourself up for failure. Expect hiccups in most adventures, so give yourself the time to be able to overcome those hurdles and still get everything you want. Ask those around you to support you and to help keep you on track with those goals as well. A "gym buddy" if you will, but for goals that are not the gym.

Are you a list person? If not, you are now. Keeping track of all your goals and plans is really going to play a factor in instant gratification here. Keep track of everything you want to do and all the things you have done already. There are apps for this but good pen to paper will do just fine. Write it all out as a list like so.

1) Order supplies
2) Paint
3) Flooring
4) New toilet
5) Wallpaper
6) Décor

As you accomplish those things, mark them off! Seeing those items lessen and getting closer to that final task is going to feel just as amazing as seeing the final product come to life. Keep a diary even. Maybe it is not a full list, but a written letter to yourself about everything you envision happening as you complete this task.

Refrain from nay-sayings. Avoid the "I can't" or "I am just not good enough". These negative thoughts will only further your lack of motivation and hold you down. I said it before and I will say it again, a win is a win no matter how small. They each need to be celebrated! So, when you get the walls painted get a coffee. When you get the décor, all purchased for your bathroom, watch your favorite movie with a friend. When you get the flowing all laid, go out to dinner. Keep track of everything as you go, so you can be prepared to make new goals as they arise or even your next task. Which room is next?

The path to get there might not be the same as everyone else. Someone on TikTok might have remodeled their bathroom in 7 days, you however are approaching day 14 with 3 more tasks. That is okay. Motivation looks different for every person as does time, money, and ability. All these factors are going to determine that path for you.

If you are mid-way through your project and you start to feel that lack of motivation, take a step back and reevaluate all that you have planned. Is your plate too full? Are the kid's schedules and workload taking much of your time right now? Is pressing pause on the project for a couple days, okay? Absolutely. Are the things on your list within your realm of ability or do you need to call in some backup? It is okay to ask for help, even if that help is someone to come paint the walls with you. Look back at your Pinterest board and remember the end goal here.

While taking a couple days to recoup is totally okay, avoid procrastination. A wise man once said, why do tomorrow what you can do today. (Within reason of course) There is a difference of taking a mental health day or having a full schedule and just putting tasks off. Procrastination is so easy to fall into. Waiting and finding distractions can instantly kill motivation. When you set up realistic goals, the timer inside of you should start. Try and race against yourself. If you have until noon to complete a task, try to get it done by 11am. That time back is going to give you time to either relax or even jump into the next tasks.

Motivation is the key to change and growth. It is going to be everything in keeping your desires on track and achieving everything you want. While you are working toward growing the power of your mind, motivation should be at the forefront of that endeavor. There will be moments when you feel like you just can't keep up or you see a lack of progress but keep pushing yourself and give yourself praise. Small steps and goals are helpful in these moments. Staying on track and motivated will sharpen your mind and really help you tap into those unbreakable thoughts.

A lack of motivation in your life is going to create anxiety and even depression. If you struggle with even the smallest of goals, you are struggling with motivation at its core, and it is not a bad idea to consider speaking to a therapist who can help you with managing your motivation.

Chapter 15: Mind Over Matter

There are many ways to use and understand mind over matter. A lot of people will use this idea or concept during intense trainings or work outs. Broken down, mind over matter is basically the ability to control physical aliments by using the mind. If you have ever seen circus performers swallow swords or lay on glass or even play with fire, it is likely they have mastered the art of mind over matter. This is important for a lot of the information you have read in this book as it shows just a bit of how powerful our thoughts really are. Understanding that power is going to be key for you to unleash it within you.

Have you ever wondered why you have a physical response to something that is more mentally stimulating? You are watching a movie, and something happens that is called a jump scare, yet your heart will race, and your palms will sweat. Nothing is there in front of you, it's a movie, but your body responds to the assumed threat, physically. All you have to do is take a deep breathe and laugh and it goes away. This is mind over matter as well. If our minds can calm down actual pain, can you imagine all the other things it can do? It is more than you know, for now. It too shall be revealed as we dive a bit further. Meditation is going to be key to finding the Zen headspace you will need to jumpstart your mind over matter journey.

Have you ever seen a video online of someone being hypnotized? Most often it is a video of someone with a soothing voice talking to a group of people or one person and the ones not talking will fall into what seems like a deep sleep, sometimes instantly. At that point the person speaking can make them think certain things or behave certain ways and they will wake to their command. Seeing this, is one way to help you understand the mind being taken over. Hypnosis has been used to help people remember their past, overcome fears, and even helped people with addiction issues. It is solid proof of just how susceptible our minds are, to a stranger. Imagine what you can achieve within your own mind.

Much like previous chapters of this book you might see another trend here. In order to get your mind ready to utilize mind over matter and overcome anything thrown at you, even pain, you are going to have to do a few key things. Exercise is one of those key things. I know, redundant but get your body moving. You will also need to get in contact with people in your life. It is shocking just how much social interaction can really play a factor in your own personal abilities. Eat right. That is not to be confused with starting a fad diet. Feed your body what it needs. Our bodies will crave what it needs if we listen to it. Our mind will do the same thing – crave what it is starving for. Start to tune into your body and your mind when it comes to cravings. Sleep. We have talked a lot about this, but it is beyond important. Set and track goals, just like when keeping motivated. Keep a journal with ideas and plans for your future. Write out what you plan to achieve while using mind over matter.

Do not underestimate your mind and all that it can do. Far too often we think "I do not have the power to do that" or "I am not like everyone else" but the fact of the matter is everyone, even you, can take advantage of the power our minds have within.

Chapter 16: Manifestation

Manifestation or the law of attraction is all about turning your dreams and thoughts into a reality. This entire book has prepared you for just this. It is the embodiment of the unbreakable thought. With the power of your mind can accomplish anything you set your mind to.

Have you ever seen someone who created a vision board? You might have laughed in the past and thought, what are they thinking? Not anymore. Those people are one step ahead of the game. They are using vision boards as a means to manifestation. Visualization is a great tool to manifest your dreams and really might be the best option to get there.

Your thoughts can control what is to come. Have you ever heard someone say the phrase, "when it rains or pours."? Hearing that might make you roll your eyes but in some regard it is true. The person who says that after one little slip up is creating a cycle or black cloud around themselves. The negative thoughts of "it can't get much worse" is going to make it get much worse immediately. They are creating the pour that is coming when it is only just raining. They are making one bad moment worse and might even be dragging it out longer than it would have been if they had remained strong and steadfast with their goals. If this is something you have been doing, it is time to stop and to shift the storyline. Instead try "this bad moment will pass" or better yet, "one moment of hard will bring 10 folds of greatness".

Some other common ways to manifest if to write down desires. You can obviously make a vison board as we mentioned but if photos are not your go to, make a list! Be sure you are writing this list as if all these goals have already happened. Here are some examples,

1) I have sold 10,000 copies of my book.

2) I finished my bathroom remodel with time to start on my bedroom

3) I am financially free

4) My mind and body are completely aligned

These are written as if the goal has been accomplished. The fact that I list 4 examples was not by accident either. The power of numbers is not something that should be overlooked either. Look into numbers, times of day, colors, and even times of the month will make these manifestations that much stronger.

The first thing you are going to manifest is seeing yourself as worthy. You are worthy of all that you desire. You deserve all that you want, and it is time that you start believing that as well. You must get your mind right and be ready to believe that these things are coming to you. Everything we have talked about in this book comes back to manifestation being the unbreakable thought. Visualization and desire will be your strength and the power of your mind we have talked so much about.

Just as manifestation can bring you all the things you desire and want in the world it also has the power to do the opposite when watered. If you are not careful with your thoughts and you continue the same bad habits and cycles, you will remain in the exact same position you are working so had to get out of. If you being to think, this is not working, I cannot do this, it is taking too long, or even I am done trying, you are going to keep setting back all the progress you have made. You must see it, believe it, *know* that is it working.

Your thoughts are energy. The more power you put into something the stronger it will become. Have you ever heard the phrase "do it with everything in you". If you focus on growth and manifestation with everything in you, and take it seriously, it will come. The more you put into something, the more power it will have. You have to up the ante for yourself. Most of the thoughts we have in a day are habit and routine. It is time to start putting energy into the thoughts you are having and redirect any of those momentary thoughts that hold us back. They will still come, but as soon as they do you should redirect them and realign your mind with your goal. You are holding yourself back by dwelling on certain things and thinking that you will never get out of this rut. You must let go of the negative manifestations in order to fill that with all the positive things you are attempting to attract.

One of the main keys to success is to see yourself as successful now. Envision the house, the car, the money, the business. All of it. To become everything, you want you must be everything you want. Turn off the negating thoughts and begin to really create the unbreakable thoughts that will change your life, they are already in you, it is time to start letting them be your voice and path.

Chapter 17: Conclusion

Have you connected the dots at this point? Followed the trail of breadcrumbs to see how investing in your mind, the states of mind, placebo effect, BDC, negative thoughts protecting your mind, your ego, and motivation all correlate to manifestation and the law of attraction? Have you seen the changes you need to make in order to become the most powerful version of yourself and how to keep your thoughts from ever being broken again? The law of attraction is really the key you have been searching for all this time. It is time that you take back your life and finally break the barrier that you have inside. For years you might have let things break you and your spirit, but it is finally time to face those fears, visualize your life, overcome all your obstacles, and push to be the strongest version of yourself to have ever existed. It is time that you ensure, your thoughts will never be broken again and create what you deserve with your mind.